The Health Literacy Guide to Picking Health Insurance

:

Introduction

Welcome to my second book based on Health Literacy and Health Living. I decided to write this series, which are all based on classes I teach in New York and Massachusetts, to bring this crucial information the country. The first three chapters of this book will explain a lot more about Public Health (I am a public health educator), Health Literacy, and Health in general. As more of these books are written, you will notice that these first three chapters do not really change. That is because it does not matter in what order you pick up the books, you still need this background information to understand why these are not your ordinary healthy living books.

These books are designed to start conversations—between you and your family, between you and your medical team, between you and your employer. They will provide more questions than answers because everyone has different health needs and, therefore, different answers will be the right set for you. And the answers will change over time because your health changes over time.

In the age of the internet, I will not share all my history and how I got to be here in this introduction. If you would like to know more about me as a professional, you are welcome to check out my LinkedIn page where I am listed as Karen Burhans Laing.

Again, I want to thank Alyssa Plock who has been my right hand person in getting these books edited and published. And I want to thank my husband, James Laing, who spent hours pouring over our health insurance options to get us the cheapest deals back when health insurance was much easier to deal with. He was the original creator of the Cost Comparison Chart.

In the meantime, I hope this book gets you thinking and talking. If you have questions, you are welcome to email me at info@healthliteracyforall.org, but the answers to your questions will mostly come from you. This is the essence of health literacy: your ability to make good every day decisions about your life based on your health and your experiences.

Be Healthy!

Karen Laing

Chapter 1: What is Public Health?

"Good Afternoon, My name is Karen Laing and I am a public health educator. Does anyone know what public health is?" I use this opening line in every class I teach. Unless I am teaching in a community that hires me regularly, I am usually met by blank stares and a lot of head shaking. And why would you know what public health is? It is the hidden side of the medical system. It is the prevention piece of the US healthcare system which works well for some, not at all for a few, and okay for most. Public health studies death, dying, and illnesses to help Americans to live as long as possible with minimum disability.

From the public health side of medicine, there are five areas of sub-specialties. The first is the research division, also known as epidemiology. These researchers are often found in state and federal health departments and they are the people who put out the contradictory test results, like coffee is good for you, coffee is bad for you, coffee is good for you. At this moment, research shows the drink one makes from coffee beans is good for you…as long as you don't smoke cigarettes with it, dunk donuts into it, or put tons of cream and sugar into it, and if your body can handle the caffeine that naturally occurs within the coffee bean.

The coffee research is a great example of why research is often contradictory and further studies often need to be done. Public health does not want to assume anything, it needs to prove that the core issue and not anything else is responsible for the results. So when coffee was first deemed bad for you, there had not been a close look at the research taking out the effects of having a cigarette with your coffee. Cigarettes have been proven over and over again to be horrible little sticks of destruction, and once the results separated out the coffee-only addicts vs the coffee-and-cigarette addict, coffee seemed healthier. When studies separated out those who drank coffee but paired it with highly un-nutritious food (like donuts and desserts), coffee again improved in the health realm. And again, there was a difference between those who drank their coffee black, those who only used a little flavoring, and those who liked "a little coffee with their cream and sugar." Then finally, research got to an individual level. How did *your* body process the caffeine? If you cannot handle caffeine, then coffee might be just fine for your neighbor and no good for you. Just like strawberries are great, unless you are allergic to them, then you should not eat them.

Once the statisticians in the research field are pretty sure they can link a cause and effect together, they will often send the research to the second division—public policy. This is where that research goes to creating laws to keep us safe. Fluoride in drinking water, and seat belt laws are two of the US's most well-known public health policies or laws.

The environmental health section, the third division, made a huge impact in the clean air and water acts from the 60s and 70s, as well as more recently with fracking and Legionnaire's disease prevention. While I was editing this book, Hurricane Harvey hit Houston. Houston is a city known for very few grassy areas (green space as it is called in public health.) Environmental health was already aware that the more green space there is, the healthier residents and employees tended to be. Perhaps because nature has a calming effect on people, perhaps because there is extra oxygen in the atmosphere from the plants. Now, with no green space in Houston, there is nowhere for the water to go to. Estimates are it could take up to two months before the water recedes/evaporates. I am sure the environmental public health division will be closely studying the effects on the buildings and people's health when the water floods a building and city for two months in comparison to the areas around Houston that had the same intensive rain, but had green space for the water to be absorbed into the ground. Look for public policy to start changing laws about the amount of green space needed for building in a year or so (the end of 2018.)

Biotechnology is the fourth subdivision. Current technology is studied and continuously improved upon. Oxygen tanks that were highly combustible, heavy, and very limiting to how far a senior could go with it have been replaced with oxygen concentrators that are lighter weight, have little risk of exploding and simply need to be plugged in to work. The lighter weight equipment combined with the increased safety has seriously improved the daily lives of those who need extra oxygen to live. Again, one can see the public health focus toward allowing people to live as full a life as possible despite the chronic illness with which they live.

Finally, I come to the last specialty area—social, behavioral and community health. How does public health change a large society to live healthier lives? One of the ways public health does this is through vaccine clinics in stores that make it convenient for people to be vaccinated. Or through public health educators who run trainings to help people understand their illnesses better. Since I started this book with the comment, I am a public health educator; you can see that this is my specialty. I train, less on specific diseases, but on a set of core values called "Health Literacy."

Chapter 2: What is Health Literacy?

According to the US government health literacy is, "the degree to which individuals have the capacity to obtain, process, and understand basic health information and services needed to make appropriate health decisions." In other words, it is a core set of skills you need to navigate the healthcare system (in sickness and in health), make healthy decisions at home, and (I have included) respond in a public health emergency. Health Literacy is understanding the ABCs of the healthcare system. Most public health educators teach on specific diseases, I teach on skills and knowledge that limit your understanding of those diseases.

Health literacy, like financial literacy, is a concept we are just beginning to recognize as key to a successful long life. If you do not know the basics of balancing a checkbook, you are inevitably going to bounce some checks along the way. If you do not understand the how and whys of taking medications, for example, you will make mistakes and end up potentially harming yourself or others.

In the United States, it is estimated that only 1 out of 10 Americans is proficient in health literacy skills. And when the mental health system is involved, the numbers go down to 1 out of 33 patients. The US medical system first recognized that patients were not fully health literate in the 1980s. Back then AIDS patients and Breast Cancer Patients both began demanding the right to be involved in their own care. They wanted to make decisions about treatment and lifestyle choices and when to end treatment. As doctors handed patients over the right to make decisions, they realized that not all patients could make the right decisions. Medical schools taught doctors to use "plain language," translators, and to provide education guides with pictures. While this was a good step toward better communication, it did not solve a patient's ability to ask questions and feel competent to make decisions. It changed the doctor's way of communicating, but did not improve the health literacy skills of the patients.

In 2012, I found myself studying health literacy for a college internship. I was asked to design a tool to help a poverty-based agency screen which of its clients needed training in health literacy. It did not take long to realize that since only 1 in 10 people were health literate, the answer was not to screen, but to train everyone. I then researched what was available to train on health literacy skills. Since it was 20 plus years since the US had identified the problem, I thought it would be easy to put together some trainings for the everyday patient to use. Sadly, that was not the case. The public health sector was still fighting over whether health literacy included skills or knowledge, as well as how to assess patients' abilities to navigate. As a retail trainer for years and a special education teacher to start my career, it made more sense to me to start training people and see how that improved health literacy skills. And so, I created the first health literacy training program in the country designed to teach everyone on these basic skills. I used the bits of curriculum I could find from cancer, heart disease, and diabetes education, along with my training as a researcher to read through the latest research. I wanted to find the pieces of knowledge and define the communication aspects that would help patients clearly share with their doctors about their health concerns, needs, and values.

When I started my work, only California taught directly to patients, and they taught only to low income parents who used Medicaid. By the time I was done with my internship, Florida had also developed a program under its English as a Second Language program. A year later, Minnesota began teaching to seniors. To the best of my knowledge, these states' program and mine are the only four programs focused on teaching skills directly to patients anywhere in the world even now five years after I started researching this. The rest of the country and the world is still trying to correct a patient deficit by retraining medical providers. In 2016, the agency I helped open won an Award from the New York State Public Health Association for Outstanding Leadership in Public Health for our work as health literacy advocates and trainers.

So why is it crucial that people have good health literacy skills? According to the federal report Inadequate Health Literacy A Barrier to Patient Care, patients who do not have good skills struggle unnecessarily and at a high cost. They are

1. More likely to report poor health status
2. Twice as likely to be hospitalized
3. Remain in the hospital more days per each admission
4. Have 1 more outpatient visit per year
5. Have more difficulty using metered inhalers
6. Have worse HbA1c levels (blood sugar levels)
7. More likely to make medication errors
8. Less likely to comply with recommended treatments.

As a result, they are more likely to be seriously disabled or die at an earlier age than someone with excellent health literacy skills. According to the National Action Plan to Improve Health Literacy, lack of health literacy skills costs the United State between $106 and $236 billion annually in medical bills alone, and an additional $238 billion in wasted medications. As you can see, it is important that public health get to the hard work of teaching Americans to improve their health literacy skills to help control medical expenses as we simultaneously help people live longer.

Chapter 3: What is Health?

Within the first few minutes of every presentation, I like to ask the questions, "What do you think health is?" and "Are you healthy?" Most people answer the first question with comments like, being able to do what you want; getting out of bed in a good mood; exercise; eating fruits and vegetables. In other words, we tend to think of health as a primarily physical thing with a bit of a mental health piece to it. But according to the World Health Organization, health consists of physical, mental, social and spiritual health. It is important that we look closely at all four aspects of health.

Most people have a pretty good idea of what physical health encompasses. Physical health is why one would see a medical doctor. It includes illnesses and disabilities. Each of us are born with a certain health level and for the rest of our lives, we make decisions to, hopefully help us stay that healthy or even get healthier. Exercise, enough sleep, good nutrition, avoiding bad habits, and learning to reduce stress are all included in the decisions made at home that reflect in the medical tests for issues like cholesterol, cancer, blood pressure and blood sugar levels. Seniors, in particular, find it harder and harder to think of themselves as physically healthy when their physical bodies naturally can do fewer and fewer things.

Most people have a fairly straight forward understanding of mental health, too. Right now, advocates are in a national push to change the term from mental health to behavioral health. Behavioral health includes minor problems like anxiety and grief and a general outlook on life, up to more serious issues like learning disabilities, drug and alcohol addictions, schizophrenia, and Alzheimer's disease. At any time, one's mental health can take a serious dive. For some people, it can return to normal with a little bit of help, or can lock a person in a world of confusion that is hard to escape. One in four people will have a problem with their mental health at some point in their lives, but not all the problems are long term, chronic diseases. As seniors age, their mental health tends to stabilize unless they develop some form of age-related dementia.

Social health is the aspect of health that as Americans, we often think about the least. It includes how we get along with others, as well as how others get along with us. The ability to hold a job, save for the future, make friends, raise a family, and enjoy the world are all aspects of social health. When physical health wanes in our old age, what keeps seniors happy and optimistic is their social health. Seeing their family and friends, living in a community with other seniors who are also socially healthy, having enough when they retire to make their lives easier, all offset the physical limitations of struggling to walk or hear or see as well.

Spiritual health is an area that we, as Americans, often do not discuss at all for fear of insulting others. Spiritual health is where one finds their inner strength to get through the bad moments of life. It is their personal beliefs that help them reach the end of their life feeling that they lead a purposeful life. It forms a core set of values on which people make decisions, including health choices.

Spiritual health and physical health decisions should work together to help people be at peace about what they are doing. No one should put their personal values to the side when making medical decisions. This is one of the crucial areas where health literacy training comes into place. If someone does not want to take a medication or get a blood transfusion because it violates their spiritual values, they need to be able to share that with their doctor in such a way, that the doctor looks for alternative ways to treat that patient. This is not about ignoring the disease or being non-compliant; it is about balancing all aspects of your health. The same is true of social health. Many seniors will continue treatments past the point they are comfortable with, simply to keep family members happy.

When health literacy skills and all four aspects of health are taught to seniors, they can have the end of the life they want to live. As long as they are willing to open up and explain to their doctors, families, and others, how their values and their treatments intersect to either bring them peace or restlessness. Ultimately, everyone wants to live at peace with others and with themselves. And this is why one cannot ignore one's physical health, but one must balance it with their mental, social and spiritual health: and then be able to share that information comfortably.

Chapter 4: The Insurance Company

Health Insurance is one of the most confusing parts of our health care system. It is something that we should all have, because it gives us a starting place for interactions with the medical system and some free care. Under the Affordable Care Act (which as of right now is still mostly in force), we are all covered for annual exams, mammograms, and colonoscopies. Many medications for asthma and diabetes are covered for free or almost free. Your insurance company cannot refuse to cover you because of a **pre-existing condition.** That is an illness or injury you already had before you joined their plan.

That being said... health insurance is designed to help cover *some* of the costs of using our medical system. It is not inexpensive, free access to everything, or the same from one company to the other. Just before the Affordable Care Act (ACA, Obamacare) was passed, the average cost for health insurance was $10,000 per employee for most companies, maybe more if the company had a lot of families or there were a lot of smokers employed in that industry. That's a little more than $800 per month. The ACA did bring down costs to about $600 per month in many states while improving access to health care and the free benefits listed above. For many people with the tax benefits the costs are even less. But let's not kid ourselves: that is not cheap.

One of most confusing things is that insurance is not the same from one state to the next, or even from one company to the next, which is why you must understand the specific features of your insurance.

Your insurance company has some very clear responsibilities. They must outline what they cover and what they do not cover. This information can be found online, in 100-page booklets, or by a phone call to the insurance company. Any given company may not cover certain doctors, medications, and services. In New York, car insurance companies increase your premiums if you use their services a lot. Health insurers cannot charge you more if you use the services more, so they control costs by limiting the doctors, treatments, and medications they will cover. They must cover anything that the federal or state governments require. In NYS, our government requires the coverage of some chiropractic care, and our Medicaid program (for those who are low income) is expanded as broadly as the federal government will allow.

Insurance companies also have the responsibility to refuse payment for things they said they would not pay for or to charge you more for medications and treatments that are not their preferred company. One of the things that all insurers refuse to pay for are experimental treatments. Usually, the costs are covered by the drug or treatment company while they are trying to get approval, but not always. It can be very upsetting to a parent of a child dying of cancer to hear, "no, we will not cover that treatment." However, it would be much worse for all of us if the company went bankrupt because it covered everyone's desperate measures. As businesses that are expected to pay healthcare providers (and the system depends on those payments), insurance companies need to maintain the cash flow and reserves to cover what they said they will cover. They cannot create money out of thin air.

The advantage of the insurance company is that you have help with your needs, but the coverage is limited by what the company can afford, as it must balance your needs with the needs of all the people it covers.

Chapter 5: Your Responsibilities

Just as the insurance company has rules and regulations it must follow, you must understand your role in the process. You must take the time to investigate the insurance company closely and make sure they cover all your doctors and your treatments—or that you can live with changing both. I teach this class a lot in the community just before open enrollment in New York (when everyone on the New York State of Health can change health insurance companies.)

One of my very good friends is a nurse, an expert in processing paperwork for the Family and Medical Leave Act, and a cancer survivor. When I asked if she wanted to sit in on one of my picking health insurance classes, she said no. She then proceeded to pick the cheapest option out there, figuring it would cover her follow-up trips to the cancer specialist who worked in the largest oncology (cancer) group in the area. Unfortunately for her, the company was new to the area and chose to contract only with the three local hospitals and their doctors. Now, with three hospitals and all their medical staff, they were well able to meet the needs of their clients. However, they did not contract with the large oncology group and she had to choose between seeing the doctor she trusted with her life for four years and paying all the costs, or changing doctors. She admitted to me, I guess I should have taken your class!

It is *your* responsibility to know what is and is not covered.

It is also your job to use all the **free services** available to you.
The services are free because public health has proven that if
you do these things, you will be healthier or. in the
unlikelihood of a major illness, you will catch it at an earlier
stage before it has done damage to your body. They are free
to you (the insurance company pays for all the costs) because
they save lives and save the insurance company money

Included in these free items is an annual exam with a primary
care doctor and well-child checks, exams that make sure your
child is staying healthy. In infants, well child checks are done
a few days after birth and then every few months. By two,
the appointments become a once-a-year event. Vaccines for
children are covered in full. Many adult vaccines are also
covered in full or for just a few dollars. If you are traveling
overseas and need a non-standard vaccine, they will cost you
more. Sometimes your state health department may have
the vaccine for a lower cost than going through your doctor
and insurance company.

Based on your age and family and personal history, there are
other tests that are included for free. Mammograms for
women over 40 and colonoscopies for anyone over 50 are
two such exams. Occasionally, your doctor will order a non-
standard test during your annual exam that you may have to
pay for. This is not because the doctor is trying to pad the bill;
you just have a medical history that needs an extra set of
testing. In fact, doctors have no idea about costs or whether
your insurer will pay, just so he does not factor costs into his
medical treatments. For instance, if you have a family history
of breast cancer, he may order a mammogram for a 30-year-

old woman. It's the right thing to do, but it is also going to cost you a co-pay, because it is not standard free care until you are 40.

Another responsibility you have is to use your primary care doctor before you go to the Emergency Room, Urgent Care, or see a specialist. While sometimes this seems like a waste of time, your primary care doctor knows the most about you and can often do the same things an ER can do much cheaper and often more accurately. Now, that does not mean if you get shot, are involved in a serious car accident or think you are having a heart attack, you should go to your primary care doctor. Those things require an ER trip. However, your doctor can give you an asthma treatment, order an x-ray of your foot if he thinks it is broken, and watch over your baby who has a high fever.

One of the huge issues that ties up Emergency Rooms unnecessarily is taking a child for suspected strep throat to the ER. Strep throat, while nasty and painful, can cause a high fever in a child rather suddenly. If it happens in the evening, a parent could panic and want their child seen that night. But for most children, it is safe for them to be given the pain reliever his doctor recommends and to wait until morning to see the primary doctor. So what would be the advantage of doing that?

- Your child will be not be exposed to all the additional germs that are in an ER or Urgent Care.

- Your pediatrician knows your child and has a better idea of skin color, behavior, and attitude that sometimes helps with the diagnosis.
- You are not trying to keep a sick child calm in an ER or Urgent Care for hours waiting to be seen.
- If the ER staff does not get the strep stick to the back of the throat, the test may come back negative. An ER doctor is trained to trust the test. He will look inside your child's throat, but assume that the redness and irritation he is seeing is viral, not strep and tell you to go home.
- It is less likely that your primary care doctor's staff misses the back of the throat because of more experience and the fact that your child did not wait hours to be seen
- Even if the test comes back negative, a primary care doctor is trained to trust his vision and his instincts. He may look at the redness and decide "it looks like strep" and give the antibiotic anyway.
- All in all, you will get better, faster, and often, more accurate care seeing your primary care doctor for strep than the ER doctor.

These are all reasons why you should not be in the ER for most problems. There is often no harm in waiting until the next morning to be seen and then your care is much better. If you are unsure whether to go to the ER or Urgent Care, you can always call your doctor's office. Someone will return your phone call and give you good advice on what to do.

Another requirement of using your health insurance well is to take your medications as prescribed. Failing to do so costs our country over $238 billion dollars annually in wasted medications. If you do not believe in medication, then do not take the prescription with you. Refuse it in the doctor's office and ask for an alternative option. But remember, you must do something about whatever illness took you to the doctor. You cannot simply not take medications. You must do something else to improve your health. And while there are a lot of "all-natural options" out there, all-natural does not guarantee safe. The all-natural option may have its own side effects, it may be contaminated with something else, or it may be just unhealthy. Think about it for a minute. Tobacco is all natural, as is arsenic, and rattlesnake venom. Yet we would not advocate taking those things to get healthier. Follow up with your doctor if you chose a homeopathic (all-natural) option, to be sure that you are getting better.

Finally, stop smoking. Smoking is the one behavior that will directly increase your health insurance costs. It was written into the ACA to allow the insurers to charge you more if you smoke and to pull your health insurance if you lie about it. It is considered a breach of contract to state you do not smoke when you do: even if it is only a cigarette or two a month. Cigarette use is tied to every known form of cancer and half of all cigarette smokers will die an early death. Public health professionals work so hard to prevent early deaths and cigarettes are one of our biggest concerns.

Chapter 6: Phrases that Mean MONEY

Insurance companies of all types have certain terms that relate to financial costs. Know which phrases mean money, so you know when you must spend money. When you are looking at the cost of health insurance (or any other kind of insurance) make sure you look for these words and understand how they could end up costing you.

Premium

A premium is the basic monthly or yearly cost of buying any kind of insurance. In health insurance, the premium is often paid by the company you work for, our government, or you the insured. As mentioned earlier the average premium in 2013 was about $10,000 per year per employee for most companies.

If you have a NY State of Health plan, you will pay this premium. If your income is at a certain level, you may get some of the premium you paid as a tax credit. But that will come back to you at the end of the year.

If you do not pay your premium for your health insurance, like your car insurance, you will lose your insurance.

Deductible

Once you pay your premium, you will still have to pay to use your health insurance. The deductible is the amount of money that you will have to spend before your health insurance will cover anything that is not government ordered for free. They took this concept right from your home owner's, renter's and car insurance.

Typically, the higher your premium, the lower your deductible and the higher your deductible, the lower your premium. You may have separate deductibles for medical, dental, vision, or mental health care. Or they all may be bundled into one deductible. You may also have an insurance plan that covers your medications before you meet your deductible. Or it could be that your medication costs are part of your deductible. Be sure which it is when you are picking health insurance.

Deductibles are paid directly to the providers. Remember, if you do not pay your deductible, you can have that doctor's office stop accepting you as a patient. No medical service you receive is free to the medical provider; each provider expects to receive payment for the services performed. It must either be paid by you or by the insurance company. With a high deductible, you will pay first; then the insurance company will pay once you have met the deductible.

Copays/ Co-Insurance

While deductibles are often in the $500 to $2000 range, copays and co-insurance are much smaller amounts. Co-pays are a set dollar amount for each service. They are often used for the doctor's appointment, your medication, emergency room and urgent care use. Some regular tests may also have co-pays. Co-Insurance is usually a percentage of the cost of the test or treatment. Co-insurance may also be charged if you use a doctor not in the network of regular providers. Co-insurance amounts vary from location to location.

To understand the differences, imagine that buying a gallon of milk was a covered medical expense. Your insurance might charge you $1.00 for every gallon of milk you buy, no matter where you get it from. So whether the original cost was $4.79 at a corner store, $3.89 at Stewarts or on sale at Hannaford Grocery for $2.99, you are still going to pay $1.00. With Co-insurance, you will pay a percentage of the cost. Imagine that same gallon of milk will now cost you 35% of the price. That means if you buy the milk at the corner store, you will pay $1.67, at Stewart's for $1.36, and at Hannaford for $1.05.

When President Obama first said that using his system would bring costs down, he was envisioning that more co-insurance charges in insurance plans would encourage patients to ask how much tests and medications cost. But since the prices are not easily available, patients are often unaware of the huge differences between one location and another. The medical system is the biggest area of American life where ordinary people do not know the costs of the services they use; with insurance, they rarely pay the full cost and, therefore, have not had the same need to shop around, as they would in other areas.

Most medical facilities require the upfront payment of copays and co-insurances and may refuse treatment if you do not pay them. Some will still bill you, but if you continue not to pay they will stop accepting you as a patient.

Pharmacies and test facilities also require the payment before you can take the medication home with you or they perform the test. In New York State, for example, if you have Medicaid and cannot afford your medication copayment or coinsurance, when you tell that to the pharmacist, he must let you take the medication anyway and you will not have to pay for it later.

Out of Pocket

Out of Pocket refers to the maximum amount of money you will have to spend in a year before your health insurance covers everything else you owe that year. This is usually between $4000 and $7000 dollars and is in place to prevent you from going broke should you have a catastrophic illness.

Non-participating

Non-participating refers to a provider that does not have a contract with the insurance company. Often your insurance will cover nothing from a non-participating provider and you will be stuck with the entire bill. The provider will often let you know by simply saying, "we do not take that health insurance." Some specialists, including chiropractors, physical therapists, and psychologists, may be non-participating but will only charge you a comparable rate to a normal co-pay or will bill you on a sliding scale.

Out of Network

Out of network is another term for providers who do not contract with your insurance provider, however, the insurance company usually pays a small percentage of their bills. This could be because you travel to another state and had no choice in getting medical care there, or it could be a specialty provider, like Cancer Centers of America, that is out of the network, but the work they do is so unique that the insurance company will pay for some of it.

Usual and Customary Charges (UCC)

Usual and Customary Charges is a phrase more likely used in dental and vision insurance, it means that the insurance company does not have a contract with the provider, but will pay what the industry has declared are the usual and customary charges in the area. However, there is a lot of controversy about this system, since one can seldom find any provider who actually charges those amounts. You will be responsible for paying anything above the UCC. Your insurance company can tell you what the UCC is and then you can shop around to know how much extra you will have to pay.

Formulary

Formulary is a pharmacy term for how a medication is made and what it is generally used for. There are 13,000 known ways for the human body to break down, 6,000 known surgeries and about 4,000 medications. Formulary when used by the insurance company describes which particular medications they will cover for which illnesses. Most medications were developed by one company and then other companies may make a drug that works similarly. All of these medications are in turn given a patent and distribution is expensive at first in order to pay for all the trials needed to ensure the medications work and are safe. In order to keep costs down, the insurance company may only provide access to one or two manufacturers' drugs.

Generic Medications

Generics are drugs manufactured by a company that did not spend its resources testing the medications, but simply copied the core medication formula after its patent had expired. The company that copies the medication formula uses different fillers and stabilizers, but the active working ingredients are the same. Generic medications are the cheapest way to buy a long lasting, well proven medication and insurance companies often charge the lowest co-pays for a patient who uses the generic. This is so common that most doctors just write for the generic medication initially when prescribing a drug, because they want to help you keep costs down and know that the generics work equally well. Generic medications are not available until after the medication's patent has expired. Generics are the cheapest way to get your medications.

Many companies make generics, and your insurance company will again usually only work with one or two of them. But to save your doctor from having to know all the options, the system is set up that the doctor writes the prescription using the original name of the medication (for instance, Penicillin) and then marks a box at the bottom of the script to use the generic. The pharmacist than picks the generic of the company your insurance company contracts with. You will end up with a medication bottle with a chemical name that then states it's a generic for Penicillin.

Non-formulary
Non-formulary is the term used to indicate that this is not a preferred medication by the insurance company. Depending on your insurance contract, you may have to pay a much higher copay for using non-formulary medications, or you may have to pay the entire cost.

Off-Formulary Use
Most medications are prescribed for a specific medical problem. Occasionally, the side effects of a particular medication would be reason enough to prescribe or take the medication. For instance, anti-anxiety medications (drugs that help people stay calm) are sometimes used to help people stop smoking or to lose weight. If a doctor uses a medication for its side effects instead of what it was originally designed for it is called "off-formulary use." You may have to pay a higher deductible or the full cost, if your doctor writes a prescription for the medication on an off-formulary use, even if the medication is covered as formulary for its original use. The medication is now being "as an experimental drug," and insurance companies do not cover experimental medications and treatments.

Chapter 7: Questions You Must Ask Before You Buy

Can I see the list of participating providers?

A participating provider is a medical person, treatment centers, labs, or hospitals that has a contract with your insurance company to provide care for its clients. As mentioned, you want to make sure that your favorite doctors are covered by the insurance companies you are considering using. Not only do you want to check your primary care doctor, but also any specialists you see. If you do not love your doctor or you do not have a regular one yet, this is not as much of an issue.

Besides your doctors, you also want to make sure they include in their network your local hospital, the closest urgent care centers, any specialty treatment center you might use and, if you routinely need lab work done, the labs that are close to you.

Does the insurance coverage work in areas you travel to frequently?

If you spend more than 20% of your time in a specific area (your parent's house, a vacation home, a second business location) that is not your hometown, you may want to compare how different insurance companies work in that area. You may find a certain insurance company has a strong presence in another area and you can still be seen by providers at in-network charges.

Even for occasional travel, you want to ask how they handle coverage within New York State, out of state, and out of the US. Insurance companies are required to cover all emergency care, but their policies vary for things like colds, strep throat or medication refills. Not a big deal if you are out of your house for a week, but go on a six-week vacation and you may find yourself needing care they do not qualify as an emergency.

Are my medications on your formulary list?

Medication costs for someone with a chronic illness can be the costliest part of the one's medical care. A patient may see their doctor twice a year at $25 per appointment for follow-up, but take three different medications at $15 each month every month. While your focus might be on the $50 spent at the doctor's annually, you could be missing the $45 a month you spend on drugs. If one of those drugs is suddenly costing $45 on its own, your costs could go from $45 a month to $75 a month: that is a huge difference at the end of the year.

If the insurance company does not cover all your medications, you can ask the pharmacist for a recommendation for a medication that is within that insurance company's formulary and does basically the same thing. It may take some tweaking of new medication to get the dose at the right level for you, or even a couple of different medications before you find one that works as well as the old one. You may even find that the new medication works better than the old.

What is the coverage for urgent care, physical or occupational therapy, mental health, drug and alcohol rehab and treatments, in-home care, and chiropractic care?

Every insurance company deals with these areas a little differently and again, like medical providers, do not cover every option. If you use this kind of care, make sure you understand how it works. If you have never used these services, the insurance company can help you if and when you need them .

What are the actual deductibles, copays and coinsurances? When you add them to the premiums, which is really the better value?

The more you use your health insurance, the more you may want to pay for the premium. Remember, the more you pay for the premium, the lower your deductibles, copays, and co-insurances.

Remember to add up the information and estimates for each person in your family. To help you figure out the costs and see how this works, the next page has a little chart. You will probably be judging between two or more insurance companies or levels of coverage. But for space within this book, I gave you only two comparison columns.

Costs	Insurance A	Insurance B
Premium (monthly cost X 12)		
Deductible		
*Per individual		
*Per Family		
Estimated number of primary care appts times copay or coinsurance		
Estimated number of specialist appts times copay/coinsurance cost		
Estimated number of Emergency Room visits times copay		
Planned surgeries/child births?		
Physical Therapy, etc?		
Counseling Costs--mental health, marriage, drug, educational?		
Dental Care- 2 times per year per person		
Additional dental expenses		
Orthodontia?		
Vision Care- Eye Doctor Appt		
New glasses, contacts		
Medication costs (med x copay x 12 months)		
*husband's		
*wife's		
*kids'		
TOTAL		

Chapter 8: Additional Questions to Think About

Dental Insurance

Your health insurance may or may not include dental insurance. Most medical policies include a subsection for dental insurance for kids, but very few cover them for adults. If yours does not, you can often buy dental insurance as a separate policy for just a few dollars a month. You can often get it as an add-on from your insurer, the New York State of Health website lists dental only policies, and Aflac Insurance covers dental care in some states.

Most policies have low premiums but high deductibles or copays. Usually for your premiums, you will get cleanings done twice a year, if you have kids, there will also be fluoride, x-rays, and sealants often completely covered for free. Why? For the same reason, medical insurance covers annual exams for free. It's been proven to keep the rest of the costs down.

You will need to ask about costs for things like fillings, emergency dentistry, and dental surgery. Crowns, implants, bridges and dentures are covered at varying rates. Orthodontics (braces) are often covered on a totally different insurance package as well.

Dental Care is well worth having because there are no medical doctors who do anything with gums, teeth and jaws. Emergency rooms may give a patient with an infection or an impacted tooth pain meds and maybe an antibiotic, but then you need to see an oral surgeon for true dental care and those doctors are not covered by medical insurance.

Eye/Vision Insurance

Like dental, this comes as an add-on insurance plan for most adults, while kids are more likely to have it included within the medical plan.

Things to look at for with vision plans include a list of participating providers, and how often you can see an eye doctor and how often you can get new frames or new lenses. Most vision insurance covers annual exams for a low co-pay, and then covers a percentage of your frames, and lenses *or* will cover contacts for a year. ***Most insurance companies will not pay for both contacts and glasses in the same year.*** Add-ons like anti-glare, breakage, or transitions lenses that become sunglasses at night may or may not be covered.

National medical centers

Does your insurance work with local, national or international specialty medical centers for rare illnesses? This is crucial if you have a family history of rare chronic illnesses like cancer, or if you have already been diagnosed with one and might want to seek treatment from them.

Is the insurance company easy to deal with?

You can decide this on your own, by calling up and asking these first eight questions yourself. How responsive are the sales people on the phone? If you call for information, do they get back to you within a day? Are they genuinely pleasant and seem unrushed? Does the staff on the phone use please and thank you? These things indicate that the insurance company values you as a potential client and is more likely to be good to you as an actual client too.

You can also check with your doctors' staff if they are comfortable working with that insurance company. Insurers and providers do not historically break contracts mid-year, but it can happen. Then you can be stuck with an insurance company that no longer covers your doctor.

What happens if I make a late premium payment to my health insurance company?

If you stop paying your premiums, you will be terminated from having insurance. Just like if you do not pay your car insurance premiums. But having a clear idea of what happens if you are late with your health insurance premium is important. Will you be reinstated immediately? At the beginning of the next month? Or will you have to wait to the next open enrollment?

Also, if you get seriously ill, injured on the job, or lose your job and cannot afford your insurance anymore, what happens? In New York, if you use the Exchange, this is called a life changing event and allows you to reapply for cheaper insurance including Medicaid at any time. If you lose your job and your insurance was through your employer, you can apply at the NYS Exchange but you must do so within the first month of unemployment.

Chapter 9: Medicare

At the age of 65, everyone is required to shift to Medicare. If your company provides your insurance, they will have a system to move you to Medicare. If you had Medicaid at age 64, you will become what is called Dual Eligible and have both Medicare and Medicaid. If your income drops when you retire, you may also qualify for dual eligibility. If you have serious health concerns and want to stay living at home, you can use a trust fund to shelter some of your income and move to the dual eligibility and a specialized dual program called Managed Long-Term Care Insurance.

Please check with your insurance company if they have Medicare supplemental insurance, a Medicare specialist from your county Office of the Aging. You do need to start the application process a few months before your 65th birthday, but in all honesty, because of the ongoing changes, there is no need to look at this before you are 64.

Summary from the Medicare.gov Website

Overall, Medicare covers *medically necessary* services and supplies to treat a disease or condition. If you have a Medicare Advantage Plan (Part C) you may have some different rules (restrictions on providers, pre-authorizations) but they must provide the same coverage as Original A and B. Some services may only be covered in certain settings (in a hospital but not outpatient) or for certain conditions (not everyone gets a wheelchair).

Part A - Covers Hospital care, skilled nursing facility care, nursing home care (provided custodial care is not the only care you need), Hospice, home health services.

Part B - Medically necessary services not covered in A and Preventative Services. In general Preventative Services are free provided you use a participating provider. Part B includes Clinical research, Ambulance services, Durable medical equipment (DME), Mental health (in and out patient), Getting a second opinion before surgery, Limited outpatient prescription drugs

Part C - Medicare Advantage Plans (MA) Cover part A and B together in one plan that is run by a private company. They cover everything A and B covers and may cover more. They often cover part D as well.

Part D - Primarily covers prescriptions. Each plan works on its own formulary and some plans have tiers for their costs. Plans may change their formulary or tier plans at any time, but must give you a 60-day notice, either in writing or by providing 60 days of continuing coverage under the old system when you renew.

Paying for Medicare

If you get Social Security, Railroad Retirement Board (RRB) benefits, or Civil Service benefits, your Medicare Part B (Medical Insurance) premium will get deducted from your benefit payment. If you do not get these benefit payments and you sign up for Part B, you will get a bill.

If you buy Medicare Part A (Hospital Insurance) or you owe

Part D income-related monthly adjustment amount (IRMAA), you will always get a monthly bill for your premium. There are 3 ways to pay these bills:

1. Sign up for Medicare Easy Pay, a free service that automatically deducts your premium payments from your savings or checking account each month.

2. Pay by check or money order. Mail your Medicare premium payments to the current location stated on Medicare.gov

3. Pay by credit card. Complete the bottom portion of the payment coupon on your Medicare bill and mail it to the address on Medicare.gov.

**If your premium is late, you will get a Second Notice reminding you to pay your premium. If you do not pay the premium by the due date for the Second Notice, you will get a Delinquent Notice. If you get a Delinquent Notice and you do not pay your premium by the 25th of the month, you will lose your Medicare coverage.

For questions about what Medicare generally covers http://www.medicare.gov/coverage/your-medicare-coverage.html

You can find a complete list of all Medicare providers in your area at

https://www.medicare.gov/find-a-plan/questions/home.aspx

Chapter 10: Other Resources

Supplemental Insurance Options

There are several other companies that offer supplemental insurance. AFLAC, the duck insurance, is probably the most famous of these insurance companies. They do not cover basic health insurance, but will pay a small payout if you need to use the Emergency Room or are hospitalized. Other supplemental insurances include cancer care, dental and vision. These insurances are often sold directly to employees through their Human Resources department when the business agrees to allow them access to their employee lists. You may also purchase it directly through an independent agent. On the whole, these policies cost very little monthly and can pay out enough to cover most of your co-payment amounts. It is worth exploring to see if this is a good match for your family.

New York State EPIC Program

As of 2017, this is a Drug cost subsidy plan for seniors: they must be a New York State resident age 65 or older, have an annual income below $75,000 if single or $100,000 if married, be enrolled or eligible to be enrolled in a Medicare Part D plan (no exceptions), and not be receiving full Medicaid benefits.

You can join EPIC at any time during the year. Once

enrolled, you will receive a 'Special Enrollment Period' to join a Medicare Part D drug plan You are not eligible to receive EPIC benefits until you are enrolled in a Part D drug plan. Seniors who are not eligible to join a Medicare Part D drug plan cannot join EPIC (e.g., seniors with a union/retiree drug subsidy program that is not a Part D plan, seniors without Medicare Part A or Medicare Part B). Seniors with Medicare Advantage (HMO) health insurance can only join EPIC if they have Part D drug coverage with their HMO.

Every New York State senior should check to see if they qualify. To check, Google NYS EPIC or go directly to https://www.health.ny.gov/health_care/epic/application_contact.htm

If you are financially struggling

Charity Care:

Every hospital that accepts Medicare must have a charity care program in place to help cover the costs of those who cannot afford their co-pays or deductibles or do not have insurance. Many hospitals now include within the umbrella of their organization, doctor's offices as well. Some hospitals will include their medical providers in their charity care programs and some use it strictly for the hospital and emergency room. Either way, if co-payments and deductibles are truly beyond your budget, you can ask about the charity care program. Many large doctors' offices also have a discount or forgiveness plan if you can prove low income.

NeedyMeds.org

This is an online referral agency for helping patients to find low cost or free medications, medical supplies, or providers. You can log onto their website or download and use one of their apps. They have three apps currently: NeedyMeds Drug Discount Card, NeedyMeds Alert that can help you remember to take your medications, and NeedyMeds Storylines which can help you track your health history as well.

Sailhelps.org

The Southern Adirondack Living Center, with offices in Queensbury, Ballston Spa, and Plattsburgh NY, has a unique program that I have not found anywhere else in the Capital Region or North Country of New York State. They maintain a "medical supply loan closet." You can borrow supplies from their closet for a few days up to a month. They also loan assistive technology and durable medical equipment through its TRAID/EI project. If you have a family member that needs short term use of a hospital bed, walker, wheelchair, or want to try out some adaptive technology for your developmentally disabled child before you invest it in, it is worth a phone call or email on the Sailhelps.org website. If you do not live between Plattsburgh NY and Albany NY, you can google "Independent Living Center" and your city and state to see if your local ILC offers a similar program. If it does not, you might just want to help them start one up.

Finally,

Hopefully, this book will give you a better understanding of medical insurance. Picking an insurance company is going to require looking at those Five Questions You Need to Know, no matter if you are picking an option from Medicaid, Medicare, you have choices from your employer or your state health insurance exchange. All the information contained within this book was the latest I could find as of Sept 2017 and only applies to New York State. You need to make sure the information crosses into your state if you live elsewhere. Most concepts will crossover, but some things may not. Hopefully, I have given you enough information to find the answers you need no matter where you live. I wish you the best as you choose.

Glossary of Terms and Ideas